Happy Holiday

POUNDS

A Weight Loss Plan for Losing Holiday Pounds

Ken Underhill

Table Of Contents

HAPPY HOLIDAY POUNDS

Drink Wine and Lose Weight

Introduction

I want to thank you and congratulate you for downloading the book, *Happy Holiday Pounds!*

It's no secret that when the holidays roll around, the number on the scale begins to creep up. However, there are some things that you can do to prevent this- and even if that number is bigger after the holidays than it was before, you can do something to drop those extra pounds.

This book will give you an explanation as to why we gain weight during the holidays- perhaps because our habits change? It will also give you some tips on how to keep from packing on those pounds- and what you can do if you do gain a few.

So, sit back, relax and enjoy reading! Thanks again for downloading this book, I hope you enjoy it!

Why Do We Gain Holiday Weight?

The holidays are upon us- that means weight gain! However, the good news is: you really don't have to stress out about gaining weight during the holiday season. In fact, the truth is, if you have fitness and weight loss goals in place, you definitely want to avoid stressing out.

Still, if you just can't stop worrying about gaining weight, a study by the New England Journal of Medicine (NEJM, 2000) found that Americans really don't gain a significant amount of weight from the time between Thanksgiving Day to New Year's Day. The average amount of weight gain is around one pound during the course of the holidays.

On the other hand, that doesn't change the fact that the holidays are extremely busy and full of lots of tempting treats. The combination of these two factors can make it very difficult to stick with your fitness and weight loss habits. While we know that constantly indulging ourselves in these treats and overeating can possibly lead to weight gain, there are some underlying habits that you may end up getting into during the holidays.

The holidays are the time of year when we focus on being thankful, sharing joy, and spending time with our loved ones- we don't want to take the time to focus on potential weight gain, right? Of course not! All you want to do is to be able to relax and enjoy the holidays and still be able to keep your fitness goals on track.

This section will provide some very sneaky holiday habits that could potentially derail your efforts- and should be avoided if at all possible.

1) We use the holidays as an excuse to eat more sweets.

During the holidays, we tend to keep sweets lying around- a container of candy canes here, a bowl of chocolate on our desk at work. Everywhere we look, there are sweets. Which makes it super easy to mindlessly eat. It is so easy to just walk by and grab a piece of candy or two, which makes it difficult to keep track of what you're really eating. However, you don't have to give it up completely. Instead of having the bowls of candy lying around, keep some in your desk or cabinet. If, at the end of a meal, you really feel the need to have something sweet, then have a piece of candy. So, it's fine to partake in the holiday sweets- as long as it's in moderation.

2) We use the holidays as an excuse to avoid keeping track of weight.

In many cases, when the holidays get here, we stop keeping track of our fitness goals, weight loss progress and body composition. We figure it's the holidays, it's okay to splurge a little, right? However, instead of hiding the scale until after New Year's, you should make the conscious decision to commit yourself to paying attention to your fitness and health routines year round. On the other hand, there's no reason you should obsess over your weight, but it can be helpful to keep an eye on the scale so that you can see if you need to make any changes.

3) We use the holidays as an excuse to not exercise.

Too often, when the holidays roll around, we get too "busy" to exercise- or maybe the weather is "too bad" (too cold, snow/rain, etc). However, we should not use this as an excuse to avoid exercising. You should never allow your holiday schedule, no matter how busy and full it is, to get in the way of your workout routine. Even if you don't have time to go to the gym, you can fit in a few minutes at home- and that's better than doing nothing. A simple walk up and down the stairs or down the driveway to check the mail can help keep you on track. Try using gallons of milk, for weights, while you sit in your favorite chair. Of course, as mentioned before, the important thing is to stay focused on your priorities- which should always include taking care of yourself.

4) Stress causes us to gain weight.

HAPPY HOLIDAY POUNDS

The holidays are typically a source of increased stress. After all, we have to shop and find the perfect gift- along with everyone else out there, we have to deal with those difficult family members that expect you to be at their holiday party at the drop of a hat (or worse, expect you to have one at your house!), and so much more. However, did you know that exercise can actually help you to relieve some of that stress? When you start to feel stressed, make sure you get to your workout as soon as possible and take out your frustrations on the pavement or the weights. A great plan is to exercise when you first get up in the morning, before the "busyness" of the day catches you. Also, you should know that stress can actually cause you to be more likely to catch all the little cold/flu bugs being spread around. Exercise can help to boost your immunity and keep you healthy. Make sure you're drinking plenty of water and including plenty of Vitamins C and D in your diet.

5) Not getting sufficient sleep causes weight gain.

Since we're so busy and so stressed, often during the holidays, our sleep habits suffer. Whether we're not sleeping because we have so much on our minds or we're not sleeping because we're out late at holiday parties every night- the point is, we're not getting the sleep that our body needs to restore itself. Not sleeping can cause us to be more likely to become sick, and since we don't have normal energy levels, we don't have the desire to exercise. Not getting sufficient sleep can also can have an effect on your eating habits- even after you're full, you keep eating (or eat more junk foods and drink more sodas to boost energy levels during the day).

6) Decreased activity levels cause weight gain.

During the winter months, the daylight hours are much shorter, which naturally means that we are not as physically active and brings about changes in our normal routines and habits. If you tend to be less active during these winter holidays, consider participating in seasonal sports such as hot yoga, ice skating, or others. Additionally, if you're getting your exercise outdoors, you should have a back-up plan in place in case the weather is too rough. Whatever you do, just make sure that you're getting consistent exercise.

7) Holidays tempt us to "over-sample" which causes weight gain.

Of course, the holidays are a time for baking- and who doesn't love licking the spoon of the cake or cookie batter. However, be careful when you're taste-testing while you're cooking. A bite or two, just as a quality check is perfectly fine. However, you should always be very careful that you don't let one small taste turn into a whole meal's worth of calorie content.

8) Mindless eating causes weight gain.

Of course, mindless eating can happen year round. However, it seems to be much more prevalent during the holiday season because there are so many more treats lying around. In some cases, mindless eating is a result of stress- you're distracted and you're eating just because it's there, not because you're hungry. Try to pay attention to what you're eating, when you're eating it, so that you can keep track of your caloric intake (and make sure that you work it off). A helpful way to keep track of your caloric intake is a simple food journal.

9) Treating yourself too often causes weight gain.

You go out shopping and you need a pick-me-up. Once in a while, it's perfectly fine to opt for that high-sugar, high-fat latte, or that ice cream. However, you shouldn't make it an everyday habit. Also, remember that it's fine to treat yourself with a slice of holiday pie or a holiday cookie with that latte every now and then- just not all the time.

10) Over-indulging in all available treats can cause weight gain.

There are lots of fun, festive foods everywhere during the holidays. It can be so easy to get into the habit of eating them every time they're offered because you don't want to hurt anyone's feelings- and, it is a special occasion, right? Well, the truth is, "special" treats aren't necessarily so "special" when you're eating them all the time. So, when special treats are offered, it's perfectly acceptable to be picky about what you eat and only choose those that are high quality and that you consider your favorites. For example- don't eat those squished sugar cookies your co-worker brought in (they're not that great anyway).

So, as you can see, there are several sneaky holiday habits that can cause you to pack on the pounds- even when you're committed to health and fitness the rest of the year. However, you can also see that there are some things that you can do to prevent yourself from packing on the pounds. Even if you still put on a few pounds, after combating these holiday habits, there are still ways that you can lose weight.

Why Bother With Weight Loss?

So you gained a few pounds during the holidays- big deal right? After all, does a few extra pounds REALLY hurt? Actually, according to the Centers for Disease Control (CDC, 2014), about 34.9% of adult Americans are obese. So, while it's true that a few extra pounds may not necessarily hurt anyone- it does put you at risk for gaining more weight and falling into that obese category. Some medical conditions that can be related to obesity are heart disease, stroke, diabetes, and cancer (CDC, 2014).

The following are a few reasons to lose those extra holiday pounds. If nothing else, maybe they'll help to be your motivation- especially if you're potentially facing medical problems due to your extra holiday pounds.

Extra weight could cause health problems.

One of the biggest reasons that people decide to lose weight- even those few extra holiday pounds- is that being overweight/obese can have a negative effect on your entire body. The more weight you're carrying, the greater risk you're putting yourself at developing some serious medical conditions. Some of the more serious medical conditions linked to extra weight are:

1) Sleep apnea

2) High blood pressure

3) High cholesterol

4) Arthritis

5) Type 2 diabetes

6) Some cancers

In fact, statistics show that over three million people die every year due to being overweight/obese (WHO, 2014). So, it's definitely a good idea to shed those holiday pounds instead of allowing them to keep piling on. Simply losing five to ten percent of your current body weight can greatly lower your risk of developing one of these chronic diseases.

Extra weight affects overall physical fitness.

HAPPY HOLIDAY POUNDS

In addition to having an effect on your health, having those extra pounds (or being overweight/obese) can also have a significant impact on your level of overall physical fitness. Even if you're not training to be champion of a triathlon, physical fitness still plays an important role in your life. The extra weight can cause you to have difficulty breathing, which makes even easy tasks such as walking to your mailbox or walking up a flight of stairs much more difficult than it should be.

Extra weight affects your self-confidence.

We all know that extra weight- even just a few pounds- can significantly impact overall self-confidence (especially in women). Even just a few extra pounds can make a big difference in how your clothes fit (or if they fit). Additionally, the extra weight can make you not want to socialize with your friends and family- which can lead to depression and/or anxiety.

It is common knowledge that individuals who make the effort and are successful at losing weight (and keeping it off) through a healthy eating plan and exercise routine will feel much better both emotionally and physically.

A few things to consider:

Before you get started on any weight loss program, you should speak with your physician or another medical professional in order to help you design a program that will meet any of your special needs.

Be sure that you set reasonable, realistic goals for your weight loss journey. If you don't have realistic goals, you could experience frustrations (more on that later) and setbacks that could result in you giving up, before you achieve your goals.

Remember that you're not going to lose it all overnight- it's going to take some time and patience. The next couple of chapters are going to tell you what not to do when trying to lose weight. Then, you'll learn what you should do- which is consume a healthy diet and get plenty of exercise.

Avoid Weight Loss Pills

The holidays have not been kind to you at all-you've been eating a lot more than usual and your workout routine just went right out the window since you were so busy with shopping, holiday parties, and other obligations. Now, you've gained weight and you desperately want to get rid of it- and fast!

You know that there are lots of medical options out there for losing weight quickly. However, you should also be aware that lots of them actually can cause some pretty seriously negative effects on your overall health. While it is true that losing weight quickly can help boost your self-esteem, it is also true that losing weight quickly can leave you fatigued, malnourished, and dehydrated. It can leave you looking and feeling like a shriveled up prune.

We all know the best way to lose weight is by making some changes in your eating habits and starting a really great workout program, not diet pills. Of course, we also know that these diet pills tempt us by promising to "melt off that unwanted fat." Well, this isn't too far from the truth. They really do work quite effectively for helping you to quickly drop a few pounds. However, choosing one of these methods could have some serious ramifications on your health that are much more detrimental than carrying around a few extra pounds for a little bit longer.

HAPPY HOLIDAY POUNDS

Diet pills work by altering the chemicals in your brain to decrease your appetite. They are amphetamines, which is basically a legalized form of speed. The following are a few of the "extreme" weight loss pills and the problems they can cause.

Remember that while these pills are effective for weight loss, the best way to lose weight (and keep from gaining it back) is by getting plenty of exercise on a regular basis and eating a healthy diet.

1) **Hoodia**

For many generations, Hoodia has been used in Africa to combat indigestion and other such health problems. They also figured out that it works very effectively as an appetite suppressant. Hoodia is considered to be a natural weight loss supplement and appetite suppressant. However, there seems to be a bit of debate over whether or not it is as effective as is claimed. There have only been a few studies that have proven it to work. On the other hand, there is also evidence that it can cause liver damage if it's taken over an extended period of time.

2) **Orlistat**

Orlistat works by preventing your digestive tract from absorbing fat. Of course, when you are absorbing less calories, this translates to weight loss. You take this medication three times a day, before meals- and it blocks approximately thirty percent of the fat you consume. This means the fat goes through your system without being used. However, studies have proven that this is actually not as effective as once thought. The truth is, it only offers about a thirty percent reduction in your body fat. If and when you ever stop taking the drug, you are more likely to gain the weight back. Some of the side effects caused by this drug are: gas, diarrhea, and fecal incontinence occasionally.

3) **Phentermine**

This weight loss medication has been on the market for a very long time. Phentermine works by controlling the neurotransmitters in your brain in order to cause your appetite to decrease. Therefore, you're not hungry when taking this medication, which means that you eat less. Eating less means that you lose weight, right? However, taking this drug does not mean that you can eat whatever you want and be lazy. Even when you're taking phentermine, you still must pay attention to your eating habits and workout on a regular basis. Some of the side effects of phentermine you should be aware of are an elevation of your heart rate and blood pressure, as well as possible insomnia and heart palpitations.

So, while it is true that these drugs can help you to quickly lose those extra holiday pounds, they are definitely NOT the best way to do so. The best way to lose the weight, and keep it off long-term, is by eating right and exercising. If you consume a healthy diet and are physically active, you should never have to go on one of the "fad" diets or take a pill to help you lose weight.

Avoid Surgery for Weight Loss

Chances are, you really didn't gain THAT much during the holidays. However, if you were already overweight/obese, you may be considering some of the more extreme weight loss methods for dropping those extra pounds. We've already talked about some of the more popular extreme weight loss pills and the side effects they bring along with them. For some, surgery seems to be an option- though, once again, definitely not the best option.

When considering weight loss surgeries, you should keep in mind that surgery does bring with it lots of health risks. In fact, with surgery, death is one of the potential complications- is losing that extra weight "overnight" worth potentially losing your life? Some of these weight loss surgeries include: liposuction or gastric bypass.

Liposuction

Let's take a look at what liposuction is and the potential complications it brings along with it. Liposuction is actually the most common- and the quickest- weight loss surgery. On the other hand, it is also the most traumatic. Depending on the amount of fat you're having sucked out, you'll either be given a mild sedative or be put completely out. A vacuum is used to suck the fat out of your body- bringing with it blood vessels and all. You'll have to wear compression garments for about a month or so, just to keep the swelling at bay.

As long as you don't experience any complications, you will be totally healed in around six weeks. However, when you have liposuction done, you could end up with bumpy or wavy skin, scarring, and even numbness. So, though it may be true that it's the quickest surgical way to lose weight, as in all procedures, it doesn't always go as smoothly or quickly as you'd like. Additionally, liposuction is really just to get you started- you will still need to eat healthy and get plenty of exercise in order to maintain your new weight.

Gastric Bypass

Gastric bypass surgery shrinks your stomach, which means you'll be eating less, which means you'll be losing weight, right? Of course, this particular extreme weight loss surgery is only for those that are extremely obese and must lose weight in order to turn their lives around or even to survive!

With gastric bypass surgery, the physician goes in and staples your stomach into a tiny, one-ounce pouch. Since your stomach is so small, you'll have a significant decrease in your caloric intake, which means that you'll end up losing lots of weight. On the other hand, gastric bypass surgery brings with it a host of potential complications. For example, your stomach can end up leaking after the surgery, which can

HAPPY HOLIDAY POUNDS

lead to infections in your body. You can also end up becoming malnourished due to the fact that a smaller stomach simply can't absorb the amount of nutrients that a full-sized one can.

So, you put on a few holiday pounds- surgery is probably not the answer unless you're extremely overweight/obese. Even if you do fit into that category and these surgeries are available to you, keep in mind the potential complications they bring with them- which typically far outweigh the benefits.

There are lots of natural fat burners available that won't have as many- if any- potentially life-threatening side effects. The best way to lose weight and keep it off is by making simple changes to your eating habits and your lifestyle. When you eat healthy and you exercise, you will see that you're not only losing weight- you feel better overall.

Lose Weight Naturally

As you have seen, quick weight loss can happen- if you're willing to risk the potential side effects of diet pills or surgery. Though these methods are quick, they're definitely NOT natural. The best way to lose weight is to do it naturally- all on your own. However, you should know that losing weight on your own without medical intervention does take lots of dedication and effort. Still, it can be done! Keep reading for tips on how to naturally lose weight without having to take diet pills, go through surgery, or follow one of those "fad" diets.

First of all, you must remember to stay hydrated. One of the best ways to ensure that you lose weight is by making sure that you're drinking plenty of water. By increasing your fluid intake, you feel full- and it helps to flush waste from your body. If you're trying to lose several pounds in a week or less, make sure that you're consistently drinking a gallon of water each day. Of course, remember to stay near a bathroom because you'll be having to go quite often for the first couple of days or so. However, it won't be long before your body will be used to consuming lots of water and you'll lose the bloat. On the other hand, don't think drinking more water will help you lose more weight. More than a gallon a day will actually overwork your kidneys. You should aim to drink at least 64 ounces, but no more than one gallon of water per day.

Next, you will need to increase your levels of physical activity (more on that later). Chances are, you're already aware that the harder your body works, the more calories you'll burn-right? You know that to lose weight, you need to be burning off more calories than you're consuming. So, if you want to drop a few pounds, add some cardiovascular exercise and weightlifting to your daily routine. Of course, keep in mind that doesn't mean that you need to be lifting 100 pounds or more. However, you should be able to start out using dumb bells in five pounds and slowly increase as you can. You should also use ankle weights in five pounds, but if you can't start with five, start with three. Then, slowly increase the weight as you can tolerate it. By using weights, you'll increase lean muscle mass and burn fat all at the same time.

In addition to the weight, you'll want to also do some cardiovascular exercise three to four days every week, making sure that you take a day off in between to allow your muscles time to rest. You can do exercises such as yoga or pilates on your off days. The simplest, low-impact cardiovascular exercise to do is just taking a walk.

Finally, when you are trying to lose weight, you must think about the nutritional aspect. Make sure that you limit your caloric intake according to your size and how much weight you plan on losing. Make sure that you do not drop below 1200 to 1500 calories each day. Be sure to choose nutritious foods such as fruits and veggies that are not high in fat or sugar. When losing weight, your diet shouldn't contain more than seven percent fat. The American Heart Association suggests that your diet consist of fruits, vegetables, and whole grains in order to ensure optimal heart health and nutrition (Heart.org, 2014).

Reduce Your Appetite to Lose Weight

During the holidays, there is definitely tons of food- and it can be so easy to just eat yourself into oblivion. However, that can lead to those post-holiday extra pounds- and that New Year's Resolution to lose weight (and never overeat again).

Of course, you already know that one of the key factors in losing weight is reducing your appetite, right? Well, it's also the most challenging because for some reason, when you hear the words "diet" or "weight loss," you're likely going to start craving everything in sight (and usually it's not the healthy food, but the unhealthy).

HAPPY HOLIDAY POUNDS

Here are a few tips that can help you to control/reduce your appetite and your cravings- and therefore, lose weight.

1) Instead of eating three large meals every day, eat more frequent, smaller meals. By eating every three to four hours, you're keeping yourself from getting too hungry- which means you are much less likely to gorge yourself when you do sit down for a meal. Eating more often keeps your body satisfied and keeps you from craving those things that aren't so good for you.

2) Increase your fiber intake because foods high in fiber content make you feel fuller much faster, and therefore, you'll end up eating less at meals. Fiber also sticks with you much longer, so you'll feel fuller much longer and therefore be able to have more control over your appetite. Make sure you take the time to chew each bite thoroughly in order to allow your brain time to realize when you're full.

3) Make sure that you include protein in each and every meal in order to keep those pesky cravings at bay. Foods that contain high levels of protein take longer to digest than other foods, therefore your blood sugar levels won't spike. Even if you're not a big fan of meat- don't worry- you can get proteins from

foods besides meats. Nuts and beans are an excellent source of protein.

4) As it has been said before- make sure you drink plenty of water. If you start to feel those annoying hunger pangs and feel like you're going to reach for something that's not so good for you- get a glass of water instead. If, after thirty minutes, you're still feeling those pesky hunger pangs, get a healthy snack- such as a piece of fruit or some veggies.

5) Believe it or not, caffeine is actually also quite effective at reducing your appetite. It is actually considered a natural appetite suppressant. However, make sure that you don't overdo it. After all, you are going to want to sleep at some point- you don't want to be wired all night from the caffeine.

6) When you finish a meal and you still feel a little hungry- wait a few minutes before grabbing that second helping. You need to give your body about twenty minutes to recognize that you've eaten. If you're still hungry after that time, get a second, but smaller helping.

We all know that when it comes to weight loss, one of the most challenging things is figuring out how you can control your appetite. As you can see in the above tips, it can be done;

HAPPY HOLIDAY POUNDS

however, it just takes a bit of dedication to yourself and your weight loss efforts.

Best Foods for Weight Loss

The holidays and all that food have caused you to accumulate stubborn belly fat. Don't worry, you're not alone! There are lots of people that are dealing with that- especially after the holidays. This book has been telling you about some natural ways to lose those extra holiday pounds. There are some foods you can consume to naturally burn it away without having to use one of the extreme weight loss methods such as diet pills or surgery. Natural foods don't bring with them the side effects that could potentially come with diet pills and/or surgery.

Some of the foods that can help you shed those unwanted holiday pounds include: lemon water, foods rich in Vitamin C, Omega-3 (not Omega-6) fatty acids, yogurt, and apple cider vinegar.

First of all, lemon water is great for the health of your liver. Your liver is basically like an air filter. You must keep it clean and maintain it, or it will get clogged up and not work correctly. Lemon water can help cleanse your liver. When it is functioning normally, your liver secretes a substance called bile, which breaks down the fat in your body. The lemon water thins the bile and keeps it flowing through the body, which helps to increase your body's metabolism of fat.

HAPPY HOLIDAY POUNDS

Foods that are rich in Vitamin C help to boost your immune system as well as lowering your body's cortisol levels. When your body is in a state of stress, your body releases a hormone called cortisol. Vitamin C works in your body to restore you to a state of calmness, and soothes stress. When your levels of cortisol have been lowered, your will see that your body is no longer storing fat, but is burning it instead.

Omega-3, not Omega-6, fatty acids are excellent for helping you to lose those extra holiday pounds. Omega-3 fatty acids actually work in two ways. First, they help to reduce inflammation in the body. After all, it's nearly impossible to lose weight when there is inflammation present in your body. Additionally, Omega-3 fatty acids work like Vitamin C to reduce cortisol levels in your body.

Yogurt- as well as other fermented foods- improve your body's immune system and ecosystem. Fermented foods contain probiotics, which provide your body with "good" bacteria. When you have good bacteria in your system, your body is better able to filter out the junk (which helps you to lose weight). Research has proven that most of the cells in our immune system (around 70 percent) are actually housed in our gut (HopkinsMedicine.org, 2014). So, this tells us that immunity is not only affected by a healthy diet but also by consuming foods that contain probiotics. If you notice that you're having a lot of upset stomachs, bloating, and constipation, it's typically due to the fact that you're not consuming enough probiotics- or "good" bacteria.

Finally, apple cider vinegar works great for helping you to meet your holiday weight loss goals. Apple cider vinegar contains a vast array of vitamins and minerals as well as acetic acid. The acetic acid is the active ingredient that works naturally with your body to melt away fat. When you are using apple cider vinegar to lose weight, you will see that your appetite will be under control, your body will be producing proteins that discourage fat accumulation, and your insulin levels will be normalized. The vinegar also makes your blood more alkaline, which is excellent. Normally, your body's pH should be just slightly on the alkaline end of the scale. However, stress and unhealthy habits cause it to become much more acidic. Just make sure that you're using unfiltered apple cider vinegar.

Fat Fighting Fruits

You already know that in order to lose weight, you'll need to make some modifications in your overall lifestyle, right? You're going to need to reduce your caloric intake and get more exercise. Fruits should definitely be a part of your weight loss plan. Many fruits are very high in fiber and will keep you feeling full. Additionally, fruits are naturally sweet, which means you'll be less likely to reach for those high-calorie, sugary snacks in the afternoons.

Of course, all fresh fruit is good for you, but there are some that are better than others for weight loss. So, when choosing fruits, consider the following to help you to meet your weight loss goals.

Melons and berries promote weight loss.

Berries and melons are low calorie, but high fiber, so they work well to keep you on track for your weight loss goals. One cup of fresh blueberries (my personal favorite) only has eighty-four calories, and a cup of sliced strawberries only contains fifty-four calories. A great afternoon snack would be a cup of Greek yogurt (remember, yogurt is great for your digestion) with a cup of sliced strawberries. If berries aren't your thing, you can always snack on some cantaloupe with a handful of almonds instead of taking a trip to the vending machine.

Other fruits that facilitate weight loss.

Some other fruits that are high in fiber, but low in calories (and are naturally sweet) include plums, pears, peaches, and apples. In most cases, fruits that have low calorie counts per gram contain high amounts of fiber and water. This means that these will fill you up quicker and you'll end up eating less than you would eat of the calorie-dense foods. Watermelon, for example, is actually 91 percent water!

Fruits, especially some of the above fruits, are an excellent choice to facilitate losing those holiday pounds. They are naturally sweet, and rich in fiber, while still being low in calories. So, you'll stay full and satisfied without having to reach for those sugary snacks in the afternoons.

Best Exercises for Weight Loss

If you find that you have gained- or are starting to gain- weight during the holidays (you know, that time between Thanksgiving and New Years- or for some, it begins at Halloween with all that candy!)- have no fear! There are some pretty simple exercises you can do to melt away those extra pounds.

While it is true that diet plays an essential part in any effort to lose weight, we also already know that effective exercise is an integral part of any healthy weight loss program. After all, the more calories you burn, the easier it is to create the calorie deficit that is necessary to promote weight loss.

The best exercises for weight loss will have both a cardio and a toning aspect- which allows you to see faster results, which means that you'll be more likely to stick to it. It can be very challenging to stick to an exercise program that you don't actually see working for you.

This section will outline a few exercises that will be extremely effective in your weight loss efforts. Take some time to try all of them and figure out which ones will work best for you- and the ones that you enjoy. The truth is, if you don't enjoy an exercise, even if it is effective, chances are you're not going to be willing to keep it up. Find the exercises that you'll be more likely to commit to using, on a regular basis, to shed those extra holiday pounds! Once you've found the ones that are effective for you- you'll be well on your way to that pre-holiday weight! (Or prevent yourself from gaining it in the first place!)

1) High intensity intermittent exercise, or HIIE, is effective in weight loss efforts. These exercises are defined as being short and involving alternating intense workouts with a very short rest. Sprinting is a great example of HIIE. Run as quickly as you can for about 400 meters and then take one minute- that's sixty seconds- to rest. Do this three times. Another great example of ah HIIE is tabata- this is a four minute workout that is made up of eight cycles of a 20 second workout followed by a ten second period of rest. For example, do as many squats as you possibly can in 20 seconds and then rest for ten. Then, repeat this seven more times.

2) Aerobic exercise, such as running, rowing, swimming, jumping rope, and cycling are all wonderful choices if you're trying to burn off those extra calories you're consuming during the holidays. Of course, swimming should be done indoors- you wouldn't want to get frostbite, would you? Did you know that running for one hour at a moderate, 10 minute pace will help you to burn over 500 calories? That's a lot of

calories! On the other hand, if you can't run due to an injury or if you just don't enjoy running (again, you must choose activities that you enjoy doing or you won't stick with them), rowing or cycling are excellent alternatives. In fact, if you go for a relaxed bike ride, you will burn around 250 calories per hour- and jumping rope for only twenty minutes will burn at least 200 calories- if not more! As mentioned, swimming is an excellent calorie burner- at a whopping 250 calories burned for just thirty minutes of laps.

3) While it is true that aerobic exercise will help you to burn calories, it is also important to improve your metabolism. This is the calories that your body burns naturally while at rest. To work on improving your metabolism, you're going to want to lift weights. Strength training helps to increase your lean body mass, and therefore your basal, or baseline, metabolism- which increases the amount of calories you burn both at rest and while working out- so, it's a win-win! When starting out with strength training, start with back squats and thrusts. Both of these are considered to be compound, full body movements that help to develop your overall strength as well as improve your metabolism.

4) All adults should consider walking to get in their exercise. It is inexpensive and everyone has access to it. Walking provides lots of additional health benefits including helping you to keep your weight under control. Additionally, your injury risk is much lower with walking than with most other types of exercise. In order to lose weight with walking, you should try to walk for at least 300 minutes per week (which averages out to less than an hour per day!)- or you can walk briskly for an hour five days per week. If you're already doing other exercise, you may want to consider adding a walking regimen to boost weight loss.

5) Of course, you should use interval training when you're exercising, no matter what type of exercise you're doing. This can be done by varying the pace of your exercise. For example, if you're walking- walk normally for a few minutes and then speed it up for a few. Alternate speed walking and normal walking several times. By using interval training, you are adjusting your body's aerobic system- that is, your heart rate, your metabolism, and your breathing- and you'll burn more calories as well as strengthen your muscles. While some do not consider interval training to be a type of exercise, others say that it is. After all, it does help you to see that

your body is able to naturally adapt to an increase in physical demands, which will be necessary in order to help you to reach your fitness goals.

6) Squats are excellent exercises to burn calories. After all, squats use the quads, hamstrings, and glutes- which are the largest of the muscle groups in your entire body. If you're not sure what a squat is, it is an up and down motion of the body that looks almost like getting out of a chair. Some trainers will even suggest that if you're new at doing squats, you can start out by practicing getting up and down out of a chair. If you have knee problems and you're worried about doing squats, check with your physician. However, in some cases, squatting has proven to resolve knee disorders. Make sure you do not bend your knees 90 degrees or lower.

7) Lunges are another very effective weight loss exercises. They work basically the same muscle groups as squats do, as well as some additional muscles and help to improve balance. If you're not sure how to do a lunge, simply take a large enough step that your knee forms a 90 degree angle. Make sure that you keep your spine in a neutral position- that is, upright and not bending forward. The knee of your back leg should nearly touch the floor, with your

toes taking most of your weight. Then, stand back up and switch legs.

8) Push-ups are effective weight loss exercises, as well as the classic exercise used to strengthen your core and upper body. If you're just starting out, you can start using a counter-top to push off of. Then, as you get better, you can use a bench or couch and eventually, you'll be able to do a push-up from the floor. You can also try a pushup from your floor, while on your knees. The important thing to remember with pushups is to have the correct form. Ten correct pushups are better for you than one-hundred incorrect pushups.

9) Abdominal crunches are a great exercise to help you define and strengthen your ab muscles- most commonly referred to as a "six pack," but not seen in most men or women. Experts say that there are several ways you can do crunches. You can lie on your back with your feet flat on the floor. You can lie on your back with your knees pulled towards your body and your feet not touching the floor. Many people believe that this is the best way to lose belly fat. However, the truth is, it's not. Belly fat covering up your "six pack" is actually reduced by burning more calories than you're consuming. Therefore, if you want a "six

pack," you must reduce your high-caloric food intake.

10) Finally, the bent-over row is a great exercise to help you lose weight and work out your back and biceps. Typically, this exercise is done by standing, but beginners can start out by sitting on a bench. Start out by simply making a fist and slowly add weight- you can use free weights or you can simply use two objects that are similarly shaped and weigh about the same. For example, you can use two cans of soup, two sports drinks, or even two books!

Playing Sports for Weight Loss

You know that physical activity helps you lose weight, right? Well, if you enjoy playing sports and you're trying to lose weight- you're definitely in luck! No matter what type of sports you enjoy playing- team, individual, or even alternative sports- you're definitely going to find something that can help you to reach your weight loss goals.

However, you should keep in mind that there are some sports that will be much more effective at burning fat than some of the others. So, in order to achieve the best weight loss results, you should make sure to include at least thirty minutes of some other type of physical activity in your daily routine. You can do this all at once or you can divide it up into more manageable time periods.

Of course, if you're going to play sports to lose weight, the best ones to do are those that burn large amounts of calories in short periods of time- right? As has been mentioned, the only way to lose weight is to burn more than you're consuming. One pound of fat equals 3,500 calories. Therefore, if you burn 3,500 calories, you'll end up losing one pound of fat.

Individual Sports and Weight Loss

HAPPY HOLIDAY POUNDS

If you would rather work out alone, there are several sports you can participate in that will help you to reach your weight loss goals. Did you know that a 155 pound adult, running eight miles an hour will burn approximately 950 calories per hour. Additionally, winter sports such as skiing or ice skating will burn a lot of calories. Jumping rope and rollerblading are also great individual sports to facilitate weight loss.

Team Sports and Weight Loss

Another great way to lose weight- and have fun with your friends- is team sports. The fast-paced, high activity sports are most effective for helping you to meet your weight loss goals. Some examples of these types of team sports are: tennis, football, soccer, and basketball. An adult, weighing 130 pounds will burn more than 500 calories per hour. Additionally, a 155 pound adult will burn around 844 calories per hour when participating in competitive rowing or boxing. Slower paced team sports such as baseball, volleyball, and softball also work well for burning calories, but at much slower rates. If you're interested in the more eclectic sports, try jai alai or squash- a 155 pound adult will burn around 844 calories per hour in these as well.

Alternative Sports and Weight Loss

Something you should know is that you're not limited to the traditional sports for weight loss.

HAPPY HOLIDAY POUNDS

Some of the more alternative sports can also help you to meet your weight loss goals. Martial arts burns high amounts of calories. In fact, an adult weighing 200 pounds will burn just under 1,000 calories in one hour of Tae Kwon Do. Additionally, if you enjoy being out in nature, a 154 pound adult burns around 370 pounds in one hour of a moderate hike.

Weight Loss Tips Cheat Sheet

As you have seen, there are lots of things you can do to prevent holiday weight gain- and lose it if you do end up gaining weight. Many people change their eating habits and many add exercise to their daily routine. Following is a "cheat sheet" of sorts with twenty-five things to remember about losing weight and keeping it off. These tips can help to prevent holiday weight gain and- if you end up gaining a little bit despite your best efforts- can help you to lose it.

1) Set realistic goals for weight loss. Don't expect to lose ten pounds in a week or more- even the most committed person can't do that. Set a goal of ½ pound to two pounds per week.

2) Pay attention to everything you eat. Research has proven that dieters that keep track of everything they eat end up losing twice as much as those dieters that don't. Purchase a notebook, planner, or download an app on your phone/tablet to help you keep track. There are apps that will actually calculate the calorie content for you- so you don't have to guess at how many calories you've consumed.

3) Find something to motivate you. Find a pair of jeans or dress that's too tight and

hang it where you can see it, instead of hiding it away in the closet, so that you can stay focused on your goals.

4) Ask for some help from friends and family. Everyone knows that it's much easier to accomplish your goals when you have someone who is holding you accountable to them, right? In fact, research has actually proven that those that have support from others lose more weight than those who don't.

5) Get out and get moving! Those who get physically active for two to four hours per week when trying to lose weight will end up losing more than those who live a sedentary lifestyle.

6) Monitor your portion sizes. One of the major keys to weight loss is not necessarily WHAT you're eating, but HOW MUCH of it you're eating. For example, even if you're eating chicken or fish instead of beef, if you're eating enough for three people, you're not saving calories. Following are some tips on portion sizes:

      a) 3-ounce meat/poultry/fish = the size of a deck of cards or the size of your palm

      b) 1 tsp butter/margarine = size of a postage stamp

      c) Cup popcorn, cold cereal, or berries = baseball

      d) 4-inch waffle/pancake = diameter of a CD/DVD

7) Look through your fridge and pantry and get rid of those that derail your weight loss efforts. You want to avoid those foods that tempt you- those that you mindlessly snack on just because they're there, not because you're hungry.

8) Choose ten of your favorite healthy, quick dinners and create a "dinner deck." Take some index cards and write the ingredients on one side and the directions on the other. When you can't think of anything for dinner, pick one of those cards- you know you'll like it because you've put it together, right?

9) Don't let yourself get hungry. Make sure that you eat regular meals and healthy snacks in-between. Keep some protein-rich foods on hand such as beans, chicken, tuna, and yogurt. Research has proven that foods high in protein keep you feeling fuller longer, which means you're less likely to fall prey to those high-carb snacks between meals.

10) Keep a ready supply of veggies such as cucumbers, broccoli, carrot sticks or snap peas in your fridge. When you're cooking or just want a quick snack, you

can grab those instead of a high sugar, high-carb snack.

11) Keep fruits such as apples, pears, grapes, clementines, and bananas on hand. These are easy to eat and don't require a whole lot of cutting or slicing.

12) Make some "secret" changes. You can get everyone involved in healthy eating without them even realizing it. For example, instead of whole milk, buy skim or low fat (1%) and use reduced/low-fat cream cheese and other dairy products instead of the regular full-fat versions. You can use these in recipes to save both fat and calories.

13) Get rid of the liquid calories. You may be surprised at the amount of calories that are in sodas, sweet tea, alcoholic drinks, and sports drinks. Cut those out of your diet for a serious calorie elimination. Instead, drink water flavored with cucumber, mint, lemon, or lime- and drink low fat or 1% milk instead of whole milk.

14) It can be much easier to stay committed to your weight loss goals if you allow yourself ONE treat per day (not dessert with every meal). Once a day- whether a mid-afternoon snack or an after dinner dessert, allow yourself to have one cookie or a fun-size candy bar- that's it.

This way, you won't feel deprived and splurge.

15) When you're eating a meal, pace yourself. It's not about who finishes the meal first. It's not about finishing quickly so you can get other things done. Instead, when you're eating- enjoy each and every bite. Rushing yourself doesn't allow your body time to know when it's full and you could end up sick. When you are full, it's time to stop eating.

16) Stay hydrated- especially before you eat. Take some time before you sit down for a meal to drink 16 ounces (2 glasses) of water. This can help to make you feel full, which means you'll end up eating less.

17) Instead of using the full size dishes, use smaller ones. You can fill up a smaller plate/bowl with less food and trick yourself into thinking you had a big meal. It's all about the visual cues.

18) When it comes to snacking after dinner, remind yourself that "if it's after eight, it's too late." Eating too close to bed time causes your body to store the fat rather than working it off. Never go to bed on a full stomach.

19) Experts recommend that you walk at least 10,000 steps- or about 4-5 miles, depending on the length of your stride-

per day. So, go buy yourself a pedometer and start counting your steps.

20) Occasionally, allow yourself a treat. If you're having a difficult day and are desperately craving chocolate, don't deprive yourself. Get some single serving ice creams or ice cream bars in the freezer- or consider keeping bite-sized chocolates in the freezer. That way, you have them if you're having cravings, but you must be willing to exercise self-control.

21) Never eat on the run. When it's time for a meal, sit down and eat from a plate. Don't eat while you're driving, or when you're standing at the fridge, or when you're lounging on the couch watching television. When you eat while you're distracted, you're more likely to overeat. When you go out to eat, ask for a to-go box at the beginning of the meal and go ahead and put half of it in the box to take home for the next day. If the restaurant offers bread, take one roll or breadstick from the basket and ask the server to take the rest.

22) When you're going to be eating out, take some time and figure out what you're going to eat before you get there. If you are having a salad, order the dressing on the side. Typically, restaurants will put about four tablespoons on a salad, which

equals too many calories. Dip your fork in the dressing and then take a bite of salad. You'll still have the dressing, and be consuming less calories.

23) Always make sure you get sufficient amounts of sleep. Sleep deprivation actually increases your hunger hormones and decreases the hormones that make you feel full. Additionally, being sleep deprived actually causes your body to store fat cells. All of the above can cause overeating, which leads to weight gain.

24) Successful dieters weigh themselves regularly. For some, that's every day. However, for others, that may seem a little too much. So, once a week is perfectly fine. Once you get your habits under control, once a month should be sufficient.

25) When you start meeting your goals, treat yourself. However, you shouldn't treat yourself with food. If there's something you've had your eye on: a cd/dvd, or a movie, or something else that is not food related, get it. Dieters who reward themselves end up losing more weight because the motivation is there. You could pay yourself a dollar (or other amount) for every pound you lose.

Common Weight Loss Frustrations and How to Combat Them

We all know that losing weight can be extremely frustrating, right? In fact, it has been said that frustration is actually one of the biggest dangers for those who want to lose a few pounds. You find out about a new eating/diet plan- or perhaps your physician suggests one- and you get really excited about it. However, after a few days of no results, you go right back to your unhealthy eating and fitness habits. There are some people out there who believe that nothing they do will help them to lose weight- so why do they even bother.

You should know, that everyone on a weight loss journey will end up feeling frustrated at some point in their journey. There are several common frustrations that everyone battles. However, there are some ways around these frustrations that will help you to get back on track, no matter how far off you feel you've gone.

The following are some of the most common weight loss frustrations and ways that you can overcome, or even completely avoid them.

1) "I just can't do it."

HAPPY HOLIDAY POUNDS

So, you've been going along pretty good- losing weight pretty steadily, and feeling pretty good about it. Now, you've come to a point where your weight loss has slowed down- or maybe even stopped. Now, you're quickly losing your motivation.

You should know that everyone will experience this plateau at some point in their weight loss journey. Your weight loss will suddenly stop, and you may even gain a pound or two in a week. However, you should always be patient with yourself- it's not a sprint, it's a marathon. Weight loss takes time- and if you keep at it, eventually, you will start to lose weight once again. Perhaps it's time for a little tweaking of your diet or exercise plan.

On the other hand, maybe you haven't been able to get a routine going. In this case, you need to sit down and take a look at your schedule. Try to find a time that works well for working out. If you can't get to the gym on a particular day, plan on going for an evening walk or run. This will keep your motivation up. These days, we're all so busy, it can help to have your workout written into your daily planner or to-do list. This way, it's not something you can avoid/forget- it's on the calendar.

2) You lose the weight- and it comes right back.

HAPPY HOLIDAY POUNDS

There is very little that is more frustrating when trying to lose weight, than when you're successful at losing it, but then it all comes right back. When it comes to your weight loss efforts, you should avoid being a boomerang- getting started and then stopping. Set up a workout schedule that you will be able to keep up for about two months. Then, after the two months are up, re-evaluate your schedule- you may need to find a different time that works better- or you may need to add more or even cut back on the amount of time you're working out.

3) You're losing weight- and then you plateau.

When you first get started with a new weight loss plan, the weight just seems to melt right off. You're feeling pretty good about it, right? Then- it all comes to a screeching halt. This happens to most people, believe it or not.

When this happens, you should sit down and take a look at your weight loss efforts and see if anything has changed. Perhaps you've picked up the habit of mindlessly snacking (which tends to happen quite often during the holidays). On the other hand, maybe nothing has really changed, you just need to make a change or two to get your weight loss started up again. Maybe you need to make some changes in your diet- or maybe you need to add to or make some other changes in your workout routine. There is always something you can do to get through the frustration of a plateau.

4) You get bored with the weight loss plans.

You think that if you have to even look at one more piece of fish or chicken, you'll lose your mind. Sure, you've found some really great recipes and foods- but the truth is, healthy eating and living isn't always fun. There are plenty of "blahs" that come along with it- but there are ways that you can deal with this.

For example, at the end of the week, allow yourself to have one "cheat" meal. By doing this, you can maintain your commitment to following your healthy diet the rest of the week. We're all human- when there's the possibility of a "reward" dangling in front of us, we're much more likely to be able to stay on course than if we expect ourselves to always eat healthy foods.

5) Those "trouble" zones simply won't go away.

Sure, overall, you're losing weight quite successfully. However, there are still a few parts that didn't get the weight loss memo. For men, the abdominals tend to be the most difficult to trim down. For women, the butt, hips, and thighs are typically the most troublesome.

Even though these troublesome spots are there- instead of focusing on them, focus on those things that are changing for the better. Feel good about the changes you have made rather than feeling bad about the changes that you have not been able to make.

When it comes to losing weight, we'll all feel frustrated and ready to give up at some point- so, never think you're all alone. You're going to feel at least one of the above frustrations at some point. However, be patient with yourself and work through them.

If you can't seem to get over them on your own, call a trusted friend or family member and ask for their help. Just keep up your weight loss efforts and pretty soon, you'll find the weight is melting off once again.

Why is it that avoiding frustrations can help you to lose weight more easily? In general, life goes much better when you're not stressed out and frustrated, right? **The following are a few basic tips to help you to deal with your frustrations when it comes to weight loss.**

First of all, instead of sweating the small stuff, look at the big picture. Experts say the quality of your diet is actually made up of the various choices you make over weeks and even months. Keep in mind that a healthy and successful weight loss program is not about always being perfect in everything you do- but balancing those really bad, stressful days with the good ones.

Secondly, as mentioned above, focus on the positive. Take a look at what you're doing right in your weight loss program instead of focusing on what is going wrong. So, you splurged at the office Christmas party- at least you're not doing it on a daily basis, right?

Thirdly, you will always want to keep track of your weight. No- you don't want to be obsessive about it, but observant. If you have a bad week and know that you haven't lost anything- in fact, you really believe you gained- step on the scale and find out exactly where you stand in your weight loss. If you've gained a few pounds, then simply make some adjustments to your diet and exercise routine.

Finally, as has been mentioned over and over- **ask for help**. Talk to someone about what has caused you to lose control. Was there something that happened to make you overeat one weekend or skip out on your workout? Talking to someone else can help you to gain some perspective by hearing theirs. After all, they're on the outside looking in. They can offer you some tips on how to get yourself back on track and through the frustrations of weight loss.

As we all know, frustrations are a given when it comes to losing weight. However, don't give up and don't lose hope. The truth of weight loss is this: you don't have to find a fad diet and stick to it or take diet pills in order to lose weight. Simply making some simple changes to your

HAPPY HOLIDAY POUNDS

diet/eating habits and levels of physical activity, you'll find that motivation is the key to losing the most weight.

Conclusion

Thank you again for downloading *Happy Holiday Pounds: Why We Gain Holiday Weight and How to Prevent and Lose It.*

I hope this book was able to help you to understand what happens during the holidays that derails our weight loss and fitness plans and goals. You learned what you should and shouldn't do so that you can come out of the holidays weighing what you weighed before- or even a little less!

You have learned that frustration is a given when it comes to weight loss. You may have trouble getting started and you may have trouble keeping it up after a while. However, don't lose hope- it is possible to maintain a healthy weight, you just have to put forth a little bit of effort.

The next step is to put some of these into practice. Even though it is super easy to gain weight during the holidays, with a little effort, it's just as easy to avoid gaining it in the first place. If you do happen to put on a few pounds though, don't stress yourself out over it. You can get back on track at any time.

Thank you and good luck with your weight loss and weight control goals!

HAPPY HOLIDAY POUNDS

References

American Heart Association. (2014). The American Heart Association's Diet

and Lifestyle Recommendations. *Heart.org*. Retrieved November 27, 2014 from http://www.heart.org/HEARTORG/GettingHealthy/NutritionCenter/HealthyEating/The-American-Heart-Associations-Diet-and-Lifestyle-Recommendations_UCM_305855_Article.jsp

Centers for Disease Control and Prevention. (2014). Adult Obesity Facts. CDC.gov. Retrieved November 27, 2014 from

http://www.cdc.gov/obesity/data/adult.html

Johns Hopkins Medicine. (2014). HopkinsMedicine.org. Retrieved November 27, 2014 from

http://www.hopkinsmedicine.org/integrative_medicine_digestive_center/services/nutrition_consultations.html

World Health Organization. (2014). Obesity and Overweight. Retrieved   November 27, 2014 from

http://www.who.int/mediacentre/facts heets/fs311/en/

Bonus Chapters

Eat Chocolate and Lose Weight

Drink Wine and Lose Weight

Do you have a bit of a sweet tooth- and enjoy your glass of wine at the end of the day? You probably think that you'll have to give all that up in order to lose a few pounds, right? Well, yeah- you'll definitely have to cut back. However, the good news is- you don't have to give it up all together! "Drink Wine and Look Fine." Isn't that great?! Keep reading to learn more!

Eat Chocolate and Lose Weight

Oh, I know what you're thinking: "This entire book has been focused on cutting out the junk food to lose weight. Now, you're telling me I can eat chocolate and lose weight? That's not possible!"

Bear with me though, neuroscience has shown that eating a piece of chocolate twenty minutes before a meal and five minutes after will reduce your appetite by about half. Now, you probably will not want to do this for breakfast, but doing it for your lunch and dinner would be great.

Research has shown that chocolate actually works with your body to curb those terrible sugar spikes that we get between meals. You know, shortly after a meal you just want to go crawl in bed and take a nap? The chocolate will prevent that from happening. In fact, some research has revealed that participants who had a dark chocolate bar every single day for fifteen days reduced their risk of insulin resistance by about fifty percent.

For the most part, it is the flavonoids in the dark chocolate that cause this insulin resistance reduction, dark chocolates also contain what we know as healthy fats that slow down the rate at which sugar is absorbed into your system. The slowing down of sugar absorption prevents that insulin spike. The

HAPPY HOLIDAY POUNDS

insulin spikes actually send the sugar into your fat cells, and switch off the natural fat-burning mechanisms. This causes you to feel hungry only a few hours later.

Additionally, other studies have revealed that chocolate reduces the effects of stress on your metabolism and will curb those terrible cravings you get for sweet, salty, and fatty foods you tend to get when you're stressed out.

So, yes- you can eat chocolate to facilitate weight loss. However- it must be dark chocolate- at least seventy percent cocoa. Milk chocolates and white chocolates actually contain milk- which we already know is a form of sugar. They also contain added sugar to increase the sweetness. Dark chocolate has less- if any- added sugar as well as containing monounsaturated fats and a bittersweet taste (which will make you want to eat less).

Now that you know it's okay to eat chocolate while you're trying to lose weight, you may find it quite difficult not to eat pounds of it. Researchers say that a serving size should be no bigger than the end of your thumb. If you overdo it, you could end up overloading your body with sugar and fat, as well as ruining your appetite. So, instead of eating that entire candy bar before dinner, break off a small square- moderation is key.

Just because you're trying to lose (or not gain) those holiday pounds, it's okay to eat some of

HAPPY HOLIDAY POUNDS

those holiday chocolates. Actually, believe it or not, it's much healthier to include these sweets in your diet than deprive yourself of them. Not only will allowing yourself to eat the chocolates keep you from overdoing it when you see them, the chocolate will work naturally with your body to help you eat less which can help you lose even more weight.

Drink Wine and Lose Weight

Now that your mind has been blown about eating chocolate to help you lose weight- prepare to be amazed once again: you can still have your glass of wine at the end of the day when you're trying to lose weight- especially if it's red wine. In fact, red wine is actually the best choice. **Remember this motto: "Drink Wine and Look Fine!"**

Red wines are very high in antioxidants and contain a compound known as resveratrol- which fights fat. As long as you limit yourself to one or two glasses per day, red wine can actually be part of a healthy diet- as well as assist you with your weight loss journey.

Studies have revealed that light to moderate consumption of alcohol actually lowers your risk of becoming overweight/obese. When compared with other alcoholic beverages, the results were the strongest with red wine. Results showed that drinking as many as two 5-ounce glasses of red wine each day can actually help you to maintain a healthy weight.

As mentioned, red wines contain high concentrations of resveratrol, which is a compound that is found in the skins of red grapes. This compound facilitates the breaking down of fats, which therefore reduces your body fat. Since resveratrol is breaking down your body fat, overall body fat is lowered-

HAPPY HOLIDAY POUNDS

which means that (prepare to be amazed) red wine actually causes you to lose weight!

On the other hand- you should think about this: two glasses of red wine equal 250 calories. That's more than ten percent of the daily calorie consumption of an individual on a 2,000 calorie diet. Additionally, red wine doesn't really offer any nutritional benefit and it doesn't make you feel full. So, while red wine is great for weight loss, it may not necessarily be the BEST choice you could make. Instead, opt for some red grapes if you're looking for a healthy source of resveratrol.

www.ingramcontent.com/pod-product-compliance
Lightning Source LLC
Chambersburg PA
CBHW060645290526
45793CB00001B/398